MW00881203

Intermittent Fasting 101

The Simple Science Of Achieving A Slim Body, Lose Weight And Live A Healthy & Awesome Life

Ted Duncan

Table of Contents

© Copyright 2018 by Ted Duncan - All rights reserved.

The transmission, duplication or reproduction of any of the following work including specific information will be considered an illegal act irrespective of if it is done electronically or in print.

This extends to creating a secondary or tertiary copy of the work or a recorded copy and is only allowed with express written consent from the Publisher. All additional right reserved.

The information in the following pages is broadly considered to be a truthful and accurate account of facts, and as such any inattention, use or misuse of the information in question by the reader will render any resulting actions solely under their purview.

There are no scenarios in which the publisher or the original author of this work can be in any fashion deemed liable for any hardship or damages that may befall them after undertaking information described herein. The author does not take any responsibility for inaccuracies, omissions, or errors which may be found therein.

Additionally, the information in the following pages is intended only for informational purposes and should thus be thought of as universal. As befitting its nature, it is presented without assurance regarding its prolonged validity or interim quality.

The author of this work is not responsible for any loss, damage, or inconvenience caused as a result of reliance on information as published on, or linked to, this book.

The author of this book has taken careful measures to share vital information about the subject. May its readers acquire the right knowledge, wisdom, inspiration, and success.

Introduction

Congratulations on downloading this eBook and thank you for doing so.

Intermittent Fasting (IF) is gaining quite a lot of popularity these days. You'll find more and more people switching to this kind of diet because of its effectiveness. Indeed, it is one of the most effective ways to lose weight and stay healthy. The following chapters will teach you everything there is to know about intermittent fasting:

Chapter 1 talks about the basics of intermittent fasting, this will help you build a strong foundation of what this diet is really all about.

Chapter 2 discusses the challenges you are likely to face during intermittent fasting. It also talks about how you can overcome these challenges effectively.

Chapter 3 discusses the different types of intermittent fasting. Learn about the different ways to apply the IF diet in your life.

Chapter 4 lays down the best practices you should observe before starting an intermittent fasting diet for optimal success.

Chapter 5 talks about intermittent fasting as a way of life. Unlike other diet programs out there, the IF diet is a healthy eating habit that you can safely do for life.

There are plenty of books and resources available on this subject in the market, thanks again for choosing this one! Every effort was made to ensure it is full of as much useful information as possible. Please enjoy!

If you enjoy the following content, click below to subscribe where we will send out self-improvement, non-fiction books, tips & information for you to read for FREE!

Do leave a good review as well if you found the content useful!

Click here -> http://eepurl.com/c5bzdX

Chapter 1
Intermittent Fasting 101

What Is Intermittent Fasting?

The term *intermittent fasting*, also referred as *IF*, is a kind of diet that alternates between cycles of fasting and non-fasting periods hence, it is called, *intermittent*. When you use this diet program, you will have to set a time window for eating along with a specified time period for fasting.

Also, unlike other diet programs where you are to be conscious about what you eat, intermittent fasting allows you to satisfy your sweet cravings. In fact, it does not require you to eliminate certain foods from your diet – all you have to focus on is *when* you will be eating. And yet, the diet has proven to be very effective in helping people lose stubborn fats, promoting good health.

Today, more and more people are learning and switching to the IF diet, and they could never have been happier.

But, you might be wondering: Why should I fast? Since fasting would mean going hungry for some time. So why do it? Well, various research, studies, and experiments have proven that fasting is actually good for the body. In fact, people have been fasting since ancient times.

Although, previously fasting was often resorted to for spiritual and religious reasons, today, fasting is known to be good for health. In fact, it can successfully prevent and cure plenty of diseases. By fasting even for a day, the digestive system is able to rest up, saving up energy that the body would have used for digestion. If a person does not fast, much of that energy will be spent in the digestion of food, and so the body will not be able to heal itself well.

According to the Father of Medicine, Hippocrates, there is a physician in every person, and the best way to make this physician work for you is by fasting. Indeed, fasting is a wonderful medicine that can cure a host of diseases.

There is nothing strange about fasting. Even animals fast when they are not feeling well. They use their instincts and deem it best not to eat for specific periods of time. When you practice intermittent fasting, you will avail all the benefits of fasting without having to sacrifice eating completely. Not only that, but this is also the kind of diet plan that you can use for a lifetime.

Fasting vs. Intermittent Fasting?

Unlike regular fasting where you are completely prohibited from eating for a certain period. Intermittent fasting gives you a relaxation to eat between fasting periods. Therefore, you do not need to starve yourself or worry about malnutrition. Plus, it is must easier than fasting for long periods of time and offers most of the benefits of regular fasts.

Intermittent Fasting vs. Other Diet Programs

Unlike other diet programs, intermittent fasting does not heavily focus on what you eat, it is more about *when* you eat. Of course, this does not mean that you can just stuff your face after fasting and are encouraged to make healthy food choices. Unlike other diet plans, intermittent fasting allows you to eat during your eating window.

Hence, you do not have to deprive yourself of the foods that you enjoy. Intermittent fasting can also be applied for a long period, even for a lifetime if you get the hang of it. This is very much unlike other diet programs that can only be used for a limited time because people end up losing motivation. In fact, it can be said that intermittent fasting is more of a lifestyle than a mere program that you use only when need to lose a couple of pounds.

Intermittent fasting is also easy to understand. You do not need to worry about recording your calorie intake nor do you have to do any complicated computations. In fact, if you have to compute anything at all, then it is just the number of hours for fasting and eating. This is something very simple which you can do easily. It is worth noting that the power of intermittent fasting lies in its simplicity. It lies in the power of fasting, where you intentionally stop eating for some time. It is during this period when the body activates its self-healing ability and makes you burn those stubborn fats away. Last but not the least, unlike other diet programs that can be dangerous for one's health, intermittent fasting is good for you in all kinds of aspects.

The Benefits

Intermittent fasting is well-known for having lots of benefits. Let us discuss them one by one:

- **Weight loss**

Of course, the most popular benefit of intermittent fasting is that it is very effective when it comes to weight loss. If you want to be able to shed off those stubborn fats, then IF diet can definitely do the job for you.

When it comes to losing weight, the key is to eat fewer calories than what you normally consume.

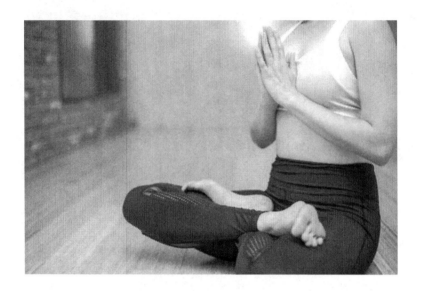

Since there will only be a limited window for eating, you will most likely consume fewer calories, which results in weight loss. Those who have tried intermittent fasting even for only a few days have experienced the powerful fat-burning benefit of this diet program.

- **Improves cell and hormone functions**

When you stop eating for a while, the body is forced to use its energy for cell repair processes. A part of this process involves removing harmful or bad substances from the cells. One's genes can also improve and promote longevity. If you want to have younger looking skin, then you should definitely try intermittent fasting.

- **Autophagy**

Autophagy is a fairly interesting process. It is known as "self-eating." When you are fasting, your body starts to utilize available stores of toxic substances or materials that are present in the body, thereby cleansing it of harmful substances. However, this is only possible when the digestive system is resting. This is why autophagy only happens when you are in a state of fasting. This is a very effective and natural way of curing diseases.

Autophagy is a wonderful benefit that can cure several ailments. Considering the bad diet and lifestyle that most people are exposed to, it is important to give your body a chance to heal and cleanse itself. Once you reach the state of autophagy, the body uses its innate ability to heal itself by removing harmful cells and substances. To reach autophagy more quickly, you can do physical exercises and try not to binge too much during your eating period.

- **Cure and prevent diseases**

Intermittent fasting can cure a host of diseases. Research shows that if you apply intermittent fasting long enough, it can prevent and even cure different kinds of diseases. This includes diabetes, high blood problems, gastrointestinal issues, and others. It is also an effective way to prevent chronic illnesses like cancer, and others.

However, for this to be possible, you also need to eat healthy foods. You cannot simply fast and then fill your stomach with unhealthy foods. Not to mention, you also need to live healthy. Therefore, avoid or quit smoking and drink with moderation.

This curative benefit of intermittent fasting primarily comes from avoiding food for certain periods of time. Since ancient times, people have fasted for healing. Even animals do not eat when they are not feeling well. Instead, they just sit still and allow the natural healing power of the body to take over. Only when they are finally healed do they start to eat normally. The same principle applies to humans. Now, you do not need to be sick to observe fasting. The practice of fasting has other benefits, such as disease prevention, cleansing the body of toxins and others.

- **Good for the heart**

Heart diseases are considered to be the world's number one killer. Fortunately, intermittent fasting has proven to be good for the heart. Fasting for certain periods of time is able to improve the risk factors associated with heart diseases. It improves cholesterol and blood triglyceride levels, as well as inflammatory markers and blood sugar levels. If only more people would learn and practice intermittent fasting, many lives would be saved.

Unfortunately, there are people who read up on IF diet, but they fail to take measures to apply this knowledge in their life. Acquiring knowledge alone is not enough. Being healthy is a way of life.

- **Good for the brain**

Studies show that intermittent fasting is good for the brain. It is also effective in preventing Alzheimer's disease and other neurodegenerative diseases. An experiment with rats also showed that intermittent fasting also helps prevent brain damage that may be caused by stroke. In the beginning, you might notice the contrary. You might feel like you cannot think clearly. Do not worry; this is quite normal when the brain is adjusting to a new diet. Just be patient, and you will soon feel the positive effects of intermittent fasting on your brain.

- **Increased focus and mental clarity**

Once you get used to intermittent fasting, you will experience increased mental focus and concentration. You will also experience a level of mental clarity that you probably have not experienced before. It is the kind of clarity that makes this diet unique. Although, this may not happen in the first few days, in fact, the first few days of fasting can be rather tough. But do not worry; this is only because your body is not yet used to your diet yet. Once your body is able to adjust to this new eating habit, you will start to experience increased focus and a state of mental clarity.

- **Boosts physical performance**

It is a common misconception that eating less or fasting will make your body weak. This will only occur at the beginning when your body is getting accustomed to your new way of life. However, once you get used to intermittent fasting, you will soon experience enhanced physical performance. This is why those who go on an intermittent fast have no problem with hitting the gym or engaging in any other physical activities.

- **Convenience**

It is worth mentioning that the IF diet is easier to follow compared to other diet programs. It is not complicated. It also does not eliminate certain foods from your diet or impose any restrictions. Instead, it only focuses on when you should eat. There is no other diet program that is simpler or more convenient than this.

- **Effective**

Without a doubt, intermittent fasting is very effective. This is why so many people are interested in learning more about this diet program. If you want to lose weight and be healthier, you will never go wrong with intermittent fasting.

- **It feels good**

After a period of fasting, your stomach will already feel cleaner. Once you start to experience the benefits of intermittent fasting, you will remain motivated. This is the first step towards leading a happier and more comfortable life.

- **Good for the skin**

Intermittent fasting is also good for your skin. It promotes cell repair and improves hormone imbalance. Intermittent fasting can beautify your skin naturally. If you suffer from skin problems like pimples or acne, intermittent fasting can significantly improve skin heath.

- **Longevity**

It is now common knowledge that intermittent fasting promotes longevity. It has been proven using many studies and experiments. So, if you want to enjoy a longer life, then this is another reason to try out intermittent fasting.

There are many other benefits of intermittent fasting. Even today, scientists are doing their best to unravel all the mysteries of this particular diet. There is no doubt that this diet program can supercharge your body and your life. Not to mention, it can also make you feel more confident, helping you succeed in life.

Can Anyone Do Intermittent Fasting?

It should be noted that although intermittent fasting is considered a very healthy diet option, it is not for everyone. If you are pregnant, suffer from eating disorders, or from any kind of serious illness, then you should double-check with a doctor.

There are conflicting views about whether a person can take up intermittent fasting during pregnancy. There is a study that suggests that IF should not be practiced by pregnant women since they need more energy for their developing baby. However, another study suggests that IF can be practiced even by pregnant women as long as they eat healthy and receive enough nutrition during the eating-window.

However, we strongly suggest pregnant women to look for an alternative way to lose weight. A better way would be to switch to IF after delivery to help shred off those stubborn belly fats.

If you have an eating disorder, then IF is definitely not for you. This is because you will require as much nutrition as you can get. The same applies if you suffer from malnutrition.

Although intermittent fasting is good for those who have diabetes and other serious diseases, you must weigh down all the risks before pursuing this diet. If you suffer from a severe illness, it is recommended you seek prior consultation from a doctor before you engage in any form of intermittent fasting.

Still, generally, it is safe to practice intermittent fasting, especially if you do not suffer from any serious disease. This is why so many people are now switching to this diet. With all the wonderful benefits that IF offers, it is definitely worth trying.

Is It Safe To Exercise?

There are many people who wonder if it is safe to exercise while on an intermittent fast. And the answer is *yes*, it is perfectly safe. After all, IF does not discourage you eating certain foods, it focuses on providing the body optimal nourishment. In this way, intermittent fasting promotes a healthier and more active life. Do not worry; you will not pass out. If you are lifting heavy weights, ensure the weights are not too heavy according to your body strength.

Even if you are not on an IF diet, it is possible to pass out when you lift something that is too heavy for you. Still, whether or not you choose to engage in strenuous exercises, intermittent fasting is definitely safe and good for you. In fact, there are many athletes and sports enthusiasts who train while following an IF lifestyle.

The Myths

Intermittent fasting also happens to be surrounded by many myths. Before you go on a full-blown IF diet, it is important you learn the truth behind these myths. This will give you a better understanding of what intermittent fasting is really all about. Let us take a look at them one by one:

- **Intermittent fasting will make you weak.**

Okay, this is a common misconception about intermittent fasting. It is only natural to experience some physical weakness during the first few days. This typically happens when you're on a low-calorie diet and the effects are only temporary. When your body finally gets used to the diet, you will start to enjoy the benefits it offers, this includes a more active lifestyle.

- **It is dangerous.**

Another common myth about IF is that it is risky and dangerous for your health. As you already know by now, intermittent fasting is actually designed to promote good health. It can even cure a host of diseases. It can only become dangerous if you do not apply it properly and deprive your body of essential nutrients for a long period of time. Given the nature and benefits of intermittent fasting, it is safe to say that more than 95% of people can safely engage in this diet without having to worry about any major side effects.

- **It can cause malnutrition.**

Malnutrition occurs when you do not feed your body essential nutrients so it can happen with any kind of diet. IF encourages folks to eat healthy foods during the eating-window and gain optimal nutrition. While it does not necessarily specify what foods should be eaten, the diet encourages you to opt for a healthy lifestyle. As long as you do not deprive your body of essential nutrients, you would not have to worry about being malnourished. In fact, you will probably be surprised to find out but human beings do not have to eat much to survive and be healthy. But of course, this is also relative to your lifestyle.

- **It is unbearable.**

If you are not used to fasting, you may find it quite unbearable in the beginning. However, the more you practice it, the more your body will adapt to it. Soon enough, you'll even find fasting for an entire day easy. You simply have to stay strong and keep trying.

- **It is still a new and untested diet program.**

Although the term intermittent fasting surfaced has only just recently, it should be noted that humans have practiced intermittent fasting for centuries. For example, back in ancient times, our ancestors had to fast due to shortage of food. Other reasons would normally involve religious customs and traditions.

However, as time went by, people began to learn more about intermittent fasting, and how it is now practiced deliberately to gain good health lose weight to look more presentable. It is also wrong to say that intermittent fasting is something that has never been tested before. Although it may be new in the sense that the term "intermittent fasting" was only developed just recently, it now has many followers.

It has been tested countless times by various people from different parts of the world, and they commend the wonderful effects and benefits of this diet.

Is It For You?

So, do you think intermittent fasting is for you? If yes, then know that this is, indeed, a wonderful diet program that can bring positive change to your life. Just imagine leading a healthier life thanks to this diet.

Still, the best way to find out and appreciate the value of intermittent fasting is by giving it a try. By the time you finish reading this book, you will be ready to go on a full-blown intermittent fast. This is something that you should be happy about as it is a very important step to a healthier and happier life. After all, being healthy is not a choice, it is an obligation that you have to your body. Understand that by becoming healthy, you can enjoy a better life.

Chapter 2
The Challenges and How To Overcome Them

Just like anything that is worth initiating, you can expect that there will be some challenges along the way. This is also true for intermittent fasting. Especially if you are just starting out, you might find some of these challenges difficult to overcome. However, do not worry; all you need is to learn the right approach and successfully overcome all obstacles that may find your way. To help prepare you even better, let us talk about certain hurdles that you will most likely face:

- **Hunger**

Hunger is the most common challenge that you will face, and you might also consider this to be one of the hardest of all challenges, especially if you are not used to staying hungry for an extended period of time. You will surely encounter hunger pangs in the beginning. Since the most important part of intermittent fasting is not eating for a certain time period, this is something that you will need to overcome.

So, how do you deal with hunger? How can you stay true to the diet when your stomach is calling out for food? Well, there are simple techniques that you can do to overcome this difficult challenge. First, you must realize that you do not need to eat, at least not yet.

The hunger that you feel only signals that your body is now trying to adjust to your new diet, which is intermittent fasting. This is actually a good sign since it means that you are making progress. Secondly, you will want to drink water. Since most people are used to eating a lot, they often confuse hunger with thirst.

Many of these hunger pangs are simply signals to remind you to drink water so drink away. Also, water can help you feel satiated. Even when you are truly hungry, drinking water can help you feel full. Not to mention, water is the best cleansing agent. When you drink water, you do not just hydrate your body, but you also wash away toxins and harmful substances in your body.

Another effective way to deal with hunger is by focusing on something else. When you are hungry, and can't think about something else, you will make things worse. So, instead of wasting your time being bothered by hunger, get busy with something and take your mind off of that feeling. It is all in the mind. If you do not focus on it, then hunger will not bother you as much.

Another thing that you can do is consider the consequences of giving in to your hunger. You will not be able to continue the intermittent fast, and you will go back to your old unhealthy way of life. Think about what that would do to your body. Is this really what you want?

You have to remind yourself that good things don't come easy. You simply have to give time to your body to adjust to your new and healthy diet. If you just give it more time and are patient enough, then you will be able to manage all those hunger pangs that you feel. Another way to deal with hunger pangs is to simply sleep on it. Hunger pangs come and go.

They are not permanent unless you continue to give them your focus and attention. Again, it is all in the mind. Last but not least, when all else fails, you simply have to exercise your willpower. This is a good time to remind yourself why you started intermittent fasting in the first place. Think about how badly you want to achieve your goals and objectives. This is all in your power. However, you will not be able to succeed if you give in to hunger. So, just stay strong as you wait for your body to adjust.

- **Mood swings**

Mood swings are very common when you are fasting. This is typically due to hunger. You may find yourself getting irritated or frustrated very easily while fasting. Hence, you are encouraged to do things that you enjoy and just be happy. You will also want to take control of your stress levels. When you are fasting, it is easier to get stressed, so try to remain calm as much as you can. If you find mood swings difficult to control, you might want to stay away from people and just have some alone time.

- **Headache**

In the beginning, when you are not quite used to fasting, you may suffer from mild headaches. Do not worry; this is normal and will go away on its own. The lesser attention you give to it, the quicker it will pass. The best way to deal with this kind of headache is by simply relaxing in bed. You can also try to just sleep it off.

- **Inconsistent weight loss**

If you want to try intermittent fasting for the purpose of losing weight, then know that IF is truly very effective. However, you might notice that the weight loss might become inconsistent over time. For example, you might lose 3 pounds in a few days only to notice that you have only lost a pound after that. However, do not worry when this happens. Again, it is just your body's way of trying to adjust to the diet. You should also consider the quality of the food that you eat during your eating window. All these things have an effect on the result of your fast.

- **It is difficult**

Although there are people who find it easy to adjust to an IF diet, there are also many who struggle to switch to intermittent fasting. Intermittent fasting can be difficult during the first few days, especially when your body isn't accustomed to staying hungry. Indeed, adjusting to a new diet can be quite difficult and bothersome. When this happens, the best thing that you can do is to stay strong and be patient as you wait for your body to finally adjust and get used to it. Thanks to our natural ability to adapt, your body will eventually find intermittent fasting easy and natural. However, before you can attain this level, you must first undergo certain challenges and wait for your body to simply get used to it.

- **Fewer meals**

Of course, a common effect of being in a state of fasting is that you will have to take fewer meals. This means that when you go out and socialize, you might have to skip eating altogether. Watching your friends eat pizza while you are fasting can definitely take a toll on your patience. Indeed, such a situation can almost be unbearable.

Well, luckily, intermittent fasting is not a strict diet. You are free to give yourself a cheat day if you want. Now, a word about cheat day: be sure to do it sparingly. If you give yourself too many cheat days, you will not be able to experience the great benefits of intermittent fasting.

Another thing that you can do, and this is the suggested approach, is to schedule your eating-window so that it coincides with your social gatherings. This way, you can be free to eat as much as you want at that moment. Of course, the best way is to still be disciplined enough to be able to resist food even when it is served in front of you but you don't necessarily have to put yourself through that situation as yet.

When you start adopting intermittent fasting, there might be situations where you would have to say *no* to the food that is on the table. Do not worry, the more that you get used to IF and appreciate its benefits, the easier it will be for you to control food cravings.

- **Tendency to binge**

Since you can only eat at a particular time, you might feel the urge to binge eat pizza and cheesy fries, along with other unhealthy foods. Now, you should keep in mind that although intermittent fasting does not have any restrictions about what you should eat, it is strongly advised that you use that time to nourish your body with healthy foods, such as vegetables and fruits.

This is important, especially if your reason for going on an IF diet is to lead a healthier lifestyle. Here, you should understand that this would require making healthy food choices. It is possible that you may be able to shred off excess fats and still be unhealthy. You should ensure that you nourish your body with adequate nutrients and stay away from unhealthy foods.

Of course, you may expect to face other challenges with hunger being the most difficult one to tackle. This is because hunger is something you feel and cannot be controlled. Your number one challenge is to overcome temptation and stop yourself from eating unhealthy.

This, of course, is not easy. This is exactly why there are people who want to be healthy but then fail to observe the IF diet. There is no secret recipe for this, except that you should just stay strong and keep on practicing. If you fail and give in to the temptation to eat, then just give it another try. Just be sure to learn from your mistake so you can avoid committing it again in the future. Simply put, you just have to stay strong and keep on trying.

You have to realize that these challenges, whatever they may be, are all part of the journey to being on an IF diet. You should not be afraid to overcome these hurdles. In fact, these challenges only signify that you are following the diet correctly. Realize that each mountain carries its own obstacles. If there are no challenges to face, then you are probably not making any progress. Therefore, instead of viewing these challenges as something bad, consider them as the essentials of living a healthy life. They are, in essence, guiding you on what to do to be healthy.

Without these challenges, it will be impossible for you to gain anything good. So, face the challenges with a positive spirit. When it comes to being successful with your diet, your state of mind is important. Hence, you should adopt a positive mindset.

These Challenges Are Good For You

It is also worth noting that experiencing these challenges is actually good and beneficial for you. These symptoms are indicators that your body is now healing itself. For example, the reason why people who are in a fasting state tend to have terrible mood swings is because their body needs to be cleansed from negativity, especially impurities.

The negative substances begin to surface and get cleaned out. So, you just have to stay strong and allow your body to do all the cleaning. Therefore, do not view these challenges as something bad, for they are essential to the healing process. As the saying goes, "No pain, no gain." You just have to hold on, and you will definitely be thankful for it soon.

By the time you have reached your eating window, you will be glad that you did not break your fast, even when you were strongly tempted to do so. You will feel cleaner, cleansed, and energized. This is the reward for sticking to the IF diet despite the challenges.

Chapter 3
Types of Intermittent Fasting

There are different ways attempt intermittent fasting. This makes the diet easier to follow. And we promise, you will not get bored with it since it is flexible enough to adapt to any kind of lifestyle. Let us now take a look at the different ways to start intermittent fasting:

16/8

The 16/8 fasting cycle is probably the most commonly used intermittent fasting cycle. What this means is that you will fast for 16 consecutive hours, and then you have an 8-hour window when you can eat. Take note that your fasting period also includes the hours you spend sleeping. Okay, this might seem so simple. You just need to fast for 16 hours, and then you have an 8-hour period to eat. Needless to say, you do not have to eat for a continuous 8 hours. This only means that within that 8-hour timeline, you can eat whatever you want. Take note, however, that to get the most benefit out of intermittent fasting, you are well advised to make healthy food choices.

Okay, let us take a closer look at this intermittent fasting model. So, you are going to fast for 16 hours. Although this might appear to be simple, it can actually be difficult to follow, especially when it is your first time. Most people are used to eating at least 3 meals a day. Not to mention, that could be three big meals, depending on how healthy you are.

There are also many who struggle just to skip a single meal, for example, dinner. If you fast for 16 hours, that is like missing out on two meals. As you can see, this can be quite challenging. But, do not worry; again, once your body is able to adjust to it, it will be very easy for you to do this 16/8 cycle.

Okay, so how can you successfully go about this diet? Instead of starting the challenge with 16 hours of fasting, start with the easy part: the 8-hour eating window. If you are just starting out, you might want to make good use of these 8 hours.

Before the 8th is over, eat something healthy that will also keep you satiated, for instance such as oatmeal. Fruits and vegetables are also excellent food choices. If you have some food cravings, it is best to eat it before the end of the 8th hour. This will allow you to completely focus on your fast.

You can expect the first few hours of the 16-hour fast to be very easy. After all, you have just eaten so won't be experiencing any hunger pangs or cravings just yet. However, you can expect to feel hungry once a few hours have passed, along with the temptation to eat. At this point, you may want to give up allow these challenges to discourage you from pursuing your fast.

However, this is also the time for you to stay strong and prove your determination. You have already been informed about this beforehand so don't allow these hurdles to catch you off guard. Just drink a glass of water and ignore your temptation to eat. Remember that you need to last up to 16 hours without food. You just have to stay strong and disciplined to stick to your diet.

While hungry, you may want time to pass quickly so that you can eat again. However, it is best you don't allow these thoughts to take control over you and divert your attention elsewhere. Instead, entertain yourself with other things. Another excellent option is to take a nap. Sleeping does not only make time fly, but it is also an effective way to suppress appetite cravings.

Just remember: No matter what happens, resist the temptation to eat. Of course, if you find yourself shaking or feeling completely unwell, then, by all means, eat something healthy. But, such events are unlikely to happen on a 16/8 intermittent fasting cycle. In fact, a 16/8 cycle is very safe, so there is nothing for you to worry about.

It is also good to remind yourself that you just need to wait for your body to adjust. The more time you give it, the easier it will become for you. If you do this long enough, then you will no longer have any problem with it. It just really takes time for the body to adjust itself to your new healthy diet. So, just think about the benefits of this diet to remain patient and calm.

23/1

The 23/1 intermittent fasting cycle is a step higher than the previous cycle. This means that you will fast for 23 hours and have an eating window of 1 hour. Once you get used to the 16/8 cycle, you can switch to a 23/1 intermittent fasting schedule. You can decide to schedule the eating period whenever you are comfortable. The important thing is to ensure that you fast for 23 consecutive hours. Again, your sleeping time is also included in your fasting period so use this to your advantage.

If you are just starting, you may be tempted to try this 23/1 challenge right away, but you will probably have a hard time with it, unless if you are already used to not eating for a long period. Unfortunately, only a few people are used to fasting, so you will most probably have a hard time surviving a 23-hour fast the first time.

Remember to be prepared because this is definitely much more challenging than the 16/8 cycle. If you want to build your pace gradually, which is also the suggested method, you might want to start with the 16/8 cycle for about 2 weeks. Once you get used to it, then you can switch to the 23/1 cycle. Do not worry; if you feel like this is too advanced for you, you can always go back to the 16/8 cycle any time you want.

Now, just because you are already used to the 16/8 cycle, it does not mean that you will only encounter a slight difficulty with the 23/1 cycle. There is a big difference between fasting for 23 hours and only 16 hours. With the 16/8 cycle, you can have several meals or snacks within 8 hours; but with the 23/1 cycle, you will most likely have only one meal, after which you will have to get back to fasting. Indeed, the 23/1 will take some preparation and getting used to. It is, however, possible, and you can do it as long as you give this diet the right preparation and commitment it requires.

By the time you the 23/1 cycle, you must have already accepted fasting as a natural part of your life. A common reason why many people are unable to fast is become they find it difficult to cope with the truths about fasting. Instead of trying to stay motivated, they keep thinking about food and more food. They are making the challenges more difficult than it actually is.

Indeed, having the right mindset is important, and an essential part of this mindset is to accept fasting as a way of life. If you do not accept this truth, then you will most likely have a hard time overcoming those hunger pangs.

So, instead of feeling sorry for yourself, remind yourself of the wonderful benefits of intermittent fasting.

Eat-Stop-Eat

This is another diet that can be used by beginners. Some people do not like the idea of eating and fasting on the same day. So, if you too feel this way, then you can use this fasting cycle instead of the 16/8 intermittent fasting cycle. When you use this method, you simply have to fast once or twice a week. You ought to fast for at least 24 hours each time.

Hence, you will have to go a whole day without eating anything. Do not worry, as you will only have to do this about two times per week.

This is a good way to prepare yourself for the real intermittent fasting journey ahead of you. Although this is also considered as intermittent fasting, it is not a full-blown diet as you can easily binge five times a week, which can ruin all your fasting efforts if you are not careful enough.

Still, this is a good beginner's fasting method to prepare yourself for a more serious and intimate IF diet. Since you can eat five days a week, it is strongly advised that you make healthy food choices. Remember that the benefits of fasting can easily be ruined by eating unhealthy foods.

This fasting method can be further developed. Once you get used to it, you can increase the number of fasting days. Instead of fasting only twice a week, you can fast three or even four times a week. This will depend on how your body adjusts to the diet. Do not forget to nourish your body with nutritious foods during eating-window days.

Alternate Day

As the name implies, alternate day fasting is when you fast alternately. For example, if you fast on a Sunday, then you will eat on Monday. You will then have to fast again on Tuesday, with an eating-window on Wednesday, then fast on Thursday, and so on. This is another healthy and powerful cycle that you can do. This is also a good cycle to use when you do not like to keep track of fasting hours. By using the alternate day fasting, all you need to do is fast today and eat tomorrow, then fast again, then eat, and so on. It is very easy to take note of.

It should be noted that you should make healthy food choices throughout this diet. Now, you might think that alternate fasting is simple and easy to do. However, it is actually more challenging than it seems. If you do it only for one or two days, then you might have no problem with it. But, once you do it for longer periods of time, you may find it incredibly challenging.

There will be times when you would want to extend the eating period. This is true, especially when you indulge yourself with lots of food during the eating-window days. Hence, it is advised that you should not binge even during the days when you can eat.

You have to train your body to be satisfied with little food and healthy foods.

Alternate day fasting is one of the best intermittent fasting cycles out there. This is definitely something that you will want to try and master. Again, it will only be hard in the beginning. Once your body gets used to it, it will become much easier. You just have to keep on practicing.

If you want to take it a step further, you can extend your fast. For example, if you start fasting today, you can end the fast tomorrow at late afternoon. The key point to remember here is that the longer you fast, the better it will be for your body. Hence, you are free to extend the fasting period when you can.

The Warrior Diet

This method is another favorite among people who practice intermittent fasting. When you are on a warrior diet, you go on a fast during the day, and then eat in the evening. By doing so, you will have enough energy recharge yourself for another fasting period the next morning. This is also a good cycle, and there are people who enjoy this method, just be careful not to binge too much every night.

If you ever feel like giving up on your diet during the day, you can simply think ahead and imagine what a wonderful evening you have ahead of you. This would be enough reason for you to stay strong and endure your diet program.

Also, since you will replenish your body with food every night, you can engage in an intense workout during the day. And since you will be recharging your system every night, you can expect to have enough energy to fast the next day.

If you don't restrict coffee from your diet, then you can drink coffee in the morning to give you that "full" feeling. Hence, the only challenge for you to overcome would be to survive your afternoon cravings. With this diet, there is always something good to look forward to every day.

Another benefit of this cycle is that you can always start fresh the next day. Since you will eat every night, you will be able to think and reflect more clearly. This will allow you to be more motivated and face another day, and this happens every single day (24 hours).

5:2 Cycle

The 5:2 diet is also known as *The Fast Diet*. According to this diet, you can eat normally for five days, but then you should dedicate two days a week for fasting. However, it would not be a strict fast. During the said two fasting days, you can still consume up to 500-600 calories. You also do not have to fast for two consecutive days. If you want, you can spread out those two days over the weekend, like Monday and Thursday. This is a matter of personal preference.

This is actually a very simple diet and is only ideal for beginners. Still, if you do not exercise and make healthy food choices especially during the 5 normal days, you will not be able to experience the real benefits of intermittent fasting. However, because of this reason, there are folks who do not consider this as a real intermittent fast. Still, it should be noted that this is an excellent beginner fasting cycle that you can use. However, do not restrict yourself to this cycle for too long. Once you start feeling more comfortable, you can switch to another more effective cycle immediately.

Feast-Fast Model

Another intermittent cycle model is known as the Feast-Fast Model. As the name implies, this is about cycling between periods of fasting and feasting. Take note, however, that the period of fasting should be longer than the period of feasting. Although it is referred to as 'feasting,' in the sense that you can eat as much as you want and anything that you like, it is not advised that you abuse it. The rule is that the more that you feast, the longer you will have to fast. Although this is also a good intermittent fasting model, it has some notable drawbacks.

For one, it might shock your digestive system if you feast after a fast. The solution here is not to feast right away but introduce foods to your body gradually. Another drawback is that that it might make your hungrier during fasting hours since you will be training your body to be very full when you feast.

It also has a strong tendency to cause people to completely binge and fall off track while eating, and this can be worse if you ever fill your stomach with unhealthy foods. It does not mean that this is not a good IF cycle, but the point here is that you should also be careful and make healthy food choices when you feast. It is also worth noting that you should not feast for more than a day. No consecutive feasts.

After a day of feasting, you should fast for more than 24 hours. This does not mean that you necessarily have to fast for 2 days. If you want, you can just fast for 35 hours or so. The important thing is to devote more time to fasting than eating. You may find it helpful to think of it in terms of hours than days.

Last but not least, this kind of cycle might not work for everyone. There are people who might end up with an upset stomach with this cycle. To know if this is for you, you will have to try it out and see for yourself. Remember to take it easy on your first try, and do not feast too much.

Spontaneous

As the term implies, this diet allows you to fast any time you want and in the same way, break the fast any time you want. Okay, this might seem like the best and easiest fast out there, but take note that this method is only as effective as the effort and dedication that you give it to. If you take it too easy on yourself, you might end up not being able to fast for a good amount of time. However, if you are disciplined and committed enough, then this might be the best intermittent fasting method for you.

For beginners, it is suggested that you start with a cycle that has a definite time period for fasting and eating. This will allow you to have a clear objective. The problem with this spontaneous method is that you can easily give in to temptation and think that you can just start all over again after eating.

The thing here is that if you keep having this kind of mindset, then you will most probably not be able to observe the right length of fasting time. In other words, you might not be able to do intermittent fasting at all, and just end up giving in to temptations. Hence, this spontaneous method is only recommended for those who already have a good experience with intermittent fasting and are truly committed to it.

When you use this method, you need to have the discipline to push yourself. You cannot just give up at the slightest temptation to break the fast and eat. Doing so will not benefit you in anyway.

Also, since you will not observe a strict cycle, it is recommended that you observe how long you fast and the length of time that you spend eating. The fasting state should not be less than 16 hours. The said 16 hours should be the minimum length of fasting. Hence, if you use this method, be sure to fast longer than 16 hours.

Make Your Own

Once you have a good deal of experience with intermittent fasting, you will be able to understand it much better. By then, you will even be able to make your own fasting cycle. The important thing is to ensure that you give time for fasting, which in no case is less than 16 hours, and then a decent window time enough for you to nourish your body with essential nutrients. Hence, you can come up with other cycles, such as 20/4, 18/6, or any other method of intermittent fasting that suits you best.

After all, there are no hard and fast rules of intermittent fasting, provided you give yourself enough time to fast on a regular basis. Regularity is important; otherwise, it would be easy for you to mess up your diet and be unhealthy.

When you make your own cycle or method, you should also consider how your body reacts to fasting, while considering your strengths and weaknesses. For example, there are people who find it easy to skip breakfast. In this case, you can fast during that time. Provided that you sleep for a couple of hours, you will easily be able to fast for 10 hours using this time frame. Of course, this will depend on how your body behaves. The point here is to use your body's behavior to make fasting more effective and efficient for you.

What Can I Consume During Fasting Period?

Unlike other fasting programs, intermittent fasting may allow you to consume beverages like coffee, tea, or even fresh juice while on a fasting state. It is worth noting, however, that this will depend on your preference. Some people only consume water while fasting, while others also consume beverages. There is only one rule to observe: the drink should have zero calories or must be a very low-calorie drink.

This can help you feel satiated instead of just drinking water. Still, if you want to take it a step further and enjoy the best benefits of intermittent fasting, it is recommended that you stick to just drinking pure and clean water when fasting. Again, this is not a strict rule. It will still depend on your personal preference and decision.

How To Break A Fast

Okay, so you have successfully survived the fasting state – what is next? Before you break your fast, there are some things that you need to know. You cannot just binge and celebrate a successful fast. You do not want to upset your stomach by shocking it with lots of food. Instead, you should warm it up gradually. It is good to break a fast by starting with something light. You might want to start it by eating soup or some vegetables. How you break your fast will also depend on the kind of body that you have.

Some people get an upset stomach if they suddenly break their fast, while others only need to start with something light and have no issues with it afterward. To be safe, always start with something light and easy for your stomach. Fruit juice is also an excellent choice. If you have fasted for more than 24 hours, then you should definitely be more careful so as not to upset your stomach. If you have no choice but to eat meat, then just eat a small amount of meat, and be sure to chew it several times in your mouth before swallowing it.

The rule is simple: start light. Avoid eating hard food, and do not eat too much. However, it is also worth noting that there are people who have no problem with breaking a fast with normal meals. After all, in intermittent fasting, you do not really fast for a long period. Still, this would depend on how long you fast, as well as how your body reacts to it.

This is something that you might want to do some trial and error on. If your stomach gets upset, then it is just a message that you should break a fast with something lighter than the meal you just had.

Combine The Cycles

If you follow the same fasting and eating period for some time, it can become boring. So, feel free to combine the different cycling periods, if you want. This way, you can benefit from a variety and prevent yourself from getting tired of the IF diet. Still, there are people who are already satisfied with just a single cycling period.

So, if you are already happy with your current diet plan, then feel free to stick to it for as long as you want. If you want some changes, then you can try other cycling periods. It is recommended that you develop your program over time. You can do this by increasing the time that you spend on fasting. The longer your fasting state is, the better it will be for your health. Of course, be sure to recharge yourself with enough nutrients during your eating window.

On Fasting

Regardless of the cycling period that you choose, it is important you learn to embrace the fasting state. After all, once you start intermittent fasting, you will find yourself fasting for long periods of time. After some time, you will begin to love the feeling of an empty and clean stomach? It just makes you feel clean and healthy. When you feel hungry (which you will), just think about the wonderful benefits of fasting, think about how your body is now able to heal itself.

The longer you stay in a fasted state, the more that you will be cleansed. You need to learn to like and appreciate the beauty of fasting. Otherwise, all those hunger pangs will appear to you as some kind of hardship instead of good signals that you are being healed. Of course, intermittent fasting is not just for healing. Fasting also works to protect and prevent you from diseases.

And, of course, the more you fast, the more you can shred off those stubborn fats. Fasting can be an amazing experience which is why many people fall in love with it. Now, you need to be careful with this. Fasting can create some kind of high. Be careful not to fast longer than you need. Remember that it is important for you to also nourish yourself with essential nutrients. Yes, you also need to eat. There are some who get so addicted to fasting that they fail to feed their body with the right amount of nutrients. So, be sure to eat right and fast properly.

When you fast, the body enjoys lots of health benefits. You may find the experience very interesting. This is good as it can help motivate you to fast even more and stick to your intermittent fasting diet.

It should also be made clear that fasting is not about going hungry without food. Hunger is just a part of fasting – and it is probably the negative part too. Think of fasting as a process of healing and detoxification. As you can see, fasting is something good and desirable. It is not something that you do to make yourself suffer. In fact, on the contrary, you can gain so much from it.

However, if you suddenly find yourself shaking or shivering or feeling sick, you should break your fast immediately. This is important to ensure safety. You should not pressure yourself too much. You do not need to learn to fast for one whole day right away. You can do it little by little until you get used to it.

Indeed, the power of fasting is incredible. This is why it is considered as a major element in intermittent fasting. It is up to you to practice it. After all, merely reading about fasting is not enough. For you to truly understand and appreciate its value, you have to put it into practice and experience it for yourself.

Vegetarianism and Intermittent Fasting

If you want to take it a step further and be truly healthy, you can safely combine being a vegetarian or a vegan with intermittent fasting. This way, you will only consume healthy foods during your eating window. It is not hard to combine the IF diet with being a vegetarian or a vegan. In fact, they complement each other and promote good health. Again, you do not have to rush things. If you want, you can do it gradually.

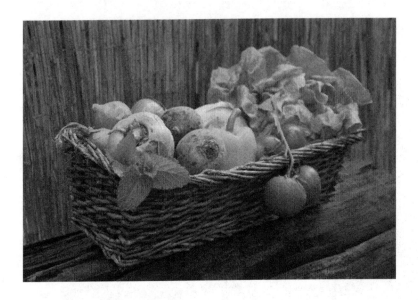

It is good to focus more on eating vegetables especially considering all the studies that advise against eating animal products which can cause inflammation and other diseases. This is another reason why you should switch to a vegan diet. It has also been proven that a person can get all their nutrition needs from vegetables alone and that there is no need to consume animal products. If you are also into the welfare of animals, then it is another good reason to go vegan. Eating lots of vegetables and intermittent fasting is a powerful way to be healthy and feel good about your body.

Chapter 4
Best Practices

Now that you know the basics about intermittent fasting, it is time you learn about certain techniques or practices that will increase your chances of success. These are practices that you should observe on a regular basis, for they can spell the difference between success and failure. Needless to say, you ought to do your best to succeed:

- **Stay Inspired**

Keep yourself inspired. It is common for people to feel motivated go on a full-blown intermittent fasting. However, after just a few days on the diet, one may be lured to temptation, wanting to eat unhealthy again. When this happens, it is only a matter of time before you finally give up and submit to the temptation. Losing your inspiration or motivation can adversely affect your willpower.

Without a strong will power, you will probably not be able to keep up with this diet for too long. So, it is important to keep your inspiration alive and remain motivated. Now, there are many ways to do this. For example, there are many videos on YouTube where people share their experiences about intermittent fasting.

You can draw inspiration by watching these videos. You can also read other books and articles on this subject. Another thing that you can do is team up with a friend. This way, you would not have to face the challenges on your own. However, be sure to pick someone who is committed enough to stick to the diet; otherwise, they might end up discouraging you. Hence, choose the right person to do this with.

Luckily, these days, it is very easy to connect with people. There are many online groups and forums that you can participate in. This is a good way to meet new people who share the same interests as yourself. This is also a good way to learn from others. If you read the posts, from time to time, you will definitely find something interesting that you can apply on your own diet. Not to mention, this is also an excellent way to make friends.

There are many ways to keep yourself inspired. However, it is also worth noting that inspiration alone is not enough. You need to be strong willed and take positive steps forward in order to succeed. There can be times when you would not feel inspired at all, such as when you are hungry, but then you need to use your willpower to stick to the diet.

- **Self-Control**

Self-control is very important if you want to follow a healthy diet. You can expect many temptations to come your way, especially when you're hungry during the fasting period. You need to be strong enough to overcome these temptations and stick to your diet regimen. When it comes to self-control, one's willpower plays an important element. You have to control yourself and the urge to abandon the diet and eat.

Now, it is worth noting that having self-control is a skill that needs to be honed. So lucky for you, this is also something that you can learn and develop. In the beginning, you might commit some mistakes. Do not be disheartened; just keep on trying. It is important that you learn to say *no* to your urges, as well as the tempting thoughts that appear in your mind. Since you are just starting out, the tendency is to be drawn to these temptations may get the better of you. Indeed, if you do not exercise self-control, you will not succeed.

When fasting, self-control is tantamount to self-restraint where you simply have to say *no* to food even when you are ravenous and have a strong urge to eat. The good news is that you can develop this skill over time. Soon enough, you will be able to restrain yourself without difficulty. In fact, you probably won't have too much of a desire to eat, especially once your body has adjusted to the IF diet. Still, self-control is very important, especially in the beginning when you are still trying to get used to the diet.

- **Listen to Your Body**

You have to learn to listen to your body. Take note that intermittent fasting is natural. Even our ancestors practiced it, although they probably didn't use the same term. You do not need any elaborate tools or equipment to do it. In fact, it is more about what you're *not doing* (not eating) than what you are doing. Listen to your body. It will also tell you when you should take a break from your fast.

This is important especially if you want to avoid health problems. For example, if you feel sick or find your body trembling, then this is certainly an indication that you should grab something to eat. Of course, common symptoms of fasting like headache, nausea, and others, can be ignored. But, if it gets too much for you to bear, then please so ahead and break your fast without guilt.

By listening to your body, you will also be able to identify your strengths and weaknesses. While intermittent fasting, you must understand how your body functions. Unfortunately, many people choose to ignore clear indicators that tell the body to slow down. Most people feel to pay attention to how their body feels, and end up reading numerous articles online, without realizing that each one of us are different from each other. By focusing on what works best for you, you will soon find yourself on the path to a healthy lifestyle.

- **Write a Journal**

Although this is not a strict requirement, many experts advise that you also use a journal. A journal will allow you to see yourself from a different perspective, from a standpoint that is free from any bias. It will also allow you to identify your strengths and weaknesses more easily. Your journal entries will act as a mirror of yourself, so it is important that you update it regularly and be as honest as you can to yourself.

To begin journal writing, you might want to use the classic pen and paper, similar to writing a diary. However, if you are not fond of *actually* writing, you might just want to use your computer. These days, you will find tons of writing applications on your mobile phone. What's best is that most of these writing applications can be downloaded for free and can be used as a journal. The important thing here is to write as regularly as you can. Moreover, you need to ensure that your file is safe and secured.

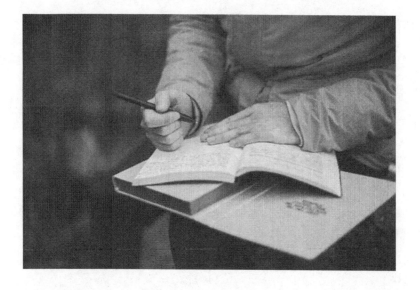

You will probably not find your journal very helpful in the first few weeks, perhaps not even in the first month. However, you are well advised to just persevere and keep on writing. After some time, especially when you are edging towards progress, you will surely start to appreciate the value and importance of writing a journal.

Okay, so what should you write in your journal, anyway? Well, since it is your own personal journal, you are free to write anything you want. You can write down your thoughts and experiences. Ideally, you can also write about your thoughts on why you chose intermittent fasting in the first place.

This can help give you a sense of direction in the future, especially when you get tempted to abandon your diet. You should also write down the mistakes that you might commit along the way so that you can avoid repeating them. Of course, you should also take note of any new knowledge that you are likely to gain in the process. Simply put, write everything in your journal that is related to your intermittent fasting experience.

It is also important to remember that a journal is not just a tool for writing; it is also for reading. In fact, it is only reading that will help you uncover many interesting lessons and points of reflection. You will find this very true when you compare your past writings with your present input. Hence, make time to reread your journal and make reflections. Indeed, having a journal can be very helpful. However, the only way for you to fully experience and appreciate its importance is to try it out and see for yourself.

- **Learn from Your Mistakes**

You should learn from your mistakes. When you first start your diet, you are likely to commit some mistakes along the way no matter how careful you may be. Do not be discouraged and hold your head up high. What is important is that you learn from your mistakes. Take the time to stop and reflect on it, and learn as much as you can. Make sure that you specify your learning of realization.

If you cannot specify it, then it only means that you have not completely understood it, so you need to spend more time reflecting. It is up to you to view these mistakes as either stumbling blocks or stepping stone that will help you become a better person. If you view each mistake in positive spirit, you will realize that each mistake is actually a lesson in disguise.

Now, do not be disheartened if you commit the same mistake several times. It only means that you need to set aside time for reflection and work on your mistakes. Be perseverant even if you are faced with failures. Again, you cannot truly be defeated unless if you stop trying.

If you are using a journal, then you should note down your mistakes, and write it down somewhere to avoid committing the same mistakes again in the future. This is where having a journal can come in handy.

While intermittent fasting, falling into temptation can be your biggest challenge. It should be noted that although this is considered normal, this is a mistake that you should avoid. This is why we have been preparing you to remain strong from the very beginning. If you fail to overcome this obstacle, then you will not be able to enjoy the benefits of intermittent fasting.

- **Live Healthy**

Although intermittent fasting does not greatly interfere with how you live your life, it is strongly advised that you follow a healthy lifestyle. If you want to be healthy and happy, then understand that you will have to do more than just fast. Being healthy is a way of life. So, if you want to enjoy the full benefits that intermittent fasting has to offer, you should also live a healthy life.

So, this is a good time for you to finally quit smoking and drinking, or at least learn to finally drink in moderation. If you have always been planning to hit the gym, now is the time for you to break some sweat and lift weights, or at least start running or do bodyweight exercises. Exercising is a natural and effective way to cleanse the body. It is also a good way to release stress and feel good.

One of the best things about intermittent fasting is that once you finally experience it, it will encourage you to live a healthy lifestyle.

Needless to say, fasting alone is not enough to make you healthy if you do not stop making unhealthy choices. One of the greatest causes of being unhealthy is stress. When you go on an IF diet, your body will already undergo stress when you fast. It is strongly encouraged that you lower your stress levels and practice mediation for increased benefits.

You do not need to change your job, but yes, you might want to start changing how you handle work, problems, and stress in general. Do not worry. Once you finally experience the beauty of being completely healthy, you will be thankful about making all these efforts. Indeed, living healthy is a great joy to experience.

- **The Right Mindset**

As the saying goes, "It is all in your mind." When you engage in intermittent fasting, you need to have the right mindset. If you do not have the right mindset, you will most probably fail. So, what does having the right mindset actually mean? Well, you need to be strong willed. If you feel like you will give up at the slightest temptation, then you will definitely fail. You need to be committed to your new way of life. You also need to be patient. As the saying goes, "Patience is a virtue."

Do not expect to be able to master intermittent fasting in just a few days. Yes, you will go hungry; yes, you will be tempted to abandon this diet. And worse, there may be times when you will even regret why you even tried intermittent fasting in the first place. However, if you stay strong and continue to just hold on a little longer, you will be very grateful for it. You should also have a strong will to succeed. So, what are your reasons for choosing this diet? You may jot down those reasons and use them to overcome your fears and obstacles.

By simply keeping these important points in mind, you will automatically feel motivated, especially during times when you already feel like giving up. Indeed, being strong willed help you in the long run.

You should also adopt a positive mindset. Take note that positive thinking is not about turning a blind eye to all the challenges you might face. That is a common misconception about positive thinking. Rather, it is more about facing challenges and obstacles with a positive spirit. Is the cup of water half full or half empty? You get to decide. Positive thinking is important to your success.

Many times, it is your own thoughts that will challenge you. You need to choose which side you are on. The only way to do this is to choose and decide to exercise positive thinking instead of being misdirected by thoughts of weakness. You need to stay strong and pursue your goal. Despite many challenges, you can overcome anything as long as remain strong and positive.

- **Do Not Overthink**

Overthinking is a common problem, especially when you are already feeling hungry. Keep in mind that although it is a good thing to keep track of your thoughts, it is not advised to overthink.

Overthinking will only make things feel worse. For example, when you experience hunger, instead of spending a lot of time thinking about it, you should just drop the thought altogether and focus on something else. This is why it can be a big advantage to learn how to control your thoughts. For this purpose, learning how to meditate can be very helpful.

When you overthink a problem or challenge, you eventually begin to feed it and give it energy. This makes the problem appear bigger or more difficult than it actually is. If you come to think about it, intermittent fasting is actually very simple and is nothing to overthink about. Overthinking will only make you feel more stressed.

So, what should you do? Well, instead of wasting your time and doubling your suffering, simply drop the idea and just try to relax. If you can, it would do you well to just sleep on it. Keep in mind that whatever challenges that you are facing are only temporary. If you can be patient enough and let time pass you by, then you will succeed. Be reminded that the power of intermittent fasting lies in its simplicity.

- **Practice Meditation**

Learning how to meditate can be very helpful when you engage in intermittent fasting. The practice of meditation has been proven to be good for one's health. It is also an effective way to reduce stress, be calm, relax, and find peace. When you feel like giving up to the challenges of intermittent fasting, sitting down even for 10 minutes in meditation can be very helpful to help you succeed.

So, what is the proper way to meditate? First, you need to learn the basics. You need to learn the proper posture. You can meditate while standing, sitting, lying, or even while walking, depending on the meditation technique you are about to use. The important thing to note here is to keep your spine straight. According to spiritual masters, there are energy centers in the body known as chakras. The chakras regulate the flow of energy in the body. Just as the physical body has its vital organs, the spiritual body has chakras.

Every person has 7 main chakras, and these chakras are located along the spine. To ensure the free flow of energy during meditation, you need to keep your spine straight.

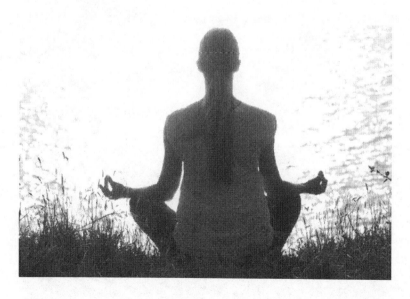

This book recommends that you meditate using a sitting position. Even the great Siddhartha Gautama Buddha achieved enlightenment while meditating in a sitting position. There are, of course, other practical reasons why you would want to meditate using a sitting position: meditating while standing or walking draws your focus on the physical body since you need to exert effort to maintain your position, although this posture is good to prevent you from falling asleep.

While lying down to meditate can be very relaxing, it can easily make you fall asleep. Meditating in a sitting position is an excellent position since you can enjoy both the benefits of having a relaxed posture, without worrying about falling asleep. This is why many people love to meditate in a sitting position. If you want, you can give these different postures a try and see for yourself.

Now that you know about the right postures, you need to understand that meditation should be made as relaxing as possible. You should not feel any pressure or exert any kind of pressure on yourself. Instead, what you need to do is simply put all your attention and focus on meditation. Many people refer to this point of focus as the mantra. Last but not least, when you meditate, especially if you are just starting, you will definitely encounter what is known as the monkey mind.

The monkey mind refers to the state of mind where your thoughts tend to jump from one branch to another like a monkey. This is where your mind jumps from one thought to another. During meditation, you might find it incredibly difficult to divert all your attention to one place. But, do not worry; you just have to keep on practicing. The more you practice, the more you will be able to control your mind.

Now that you know the important guidelines on meditation, it is time to proceed to proper meditation. The following meditation technique is known as *Meditation on the Breath*. It is a basic meditation, but it is also very effective. The steps are as follows:

1. *Assume a meditative posture and relax.*

2. *Breathe in and out gently through your nose.*

3. *Now, place all of your focus on your breathing.*

4. *Breathe in gently through the nose, and then breathe out.*

5. *If distracting thoughts arise in the mind, simply ignore them, and bring your attention back to your breath.*

6. *Relax and let go.*

The power of this meditation lies in its simplicity. If you do it properly, you might be surprised by just how powerful it is. It can give you peace of mind and harmony. When you feel like giving up on intermittent fasting, you can just sit and meditate for as long as you like and revitalize yourself.

If you enjoyed this meditation, then you might want to try the *Cleansing Breath Meditation*. The steps are as follows:

1. *Assume a meditative posture. Relax and breathe gently. With every breath, feel yourself getting more relaxed. Now, take a deep breath. As you exhale, visualize that you also exhaling all the negativity from your body. See and feel all the stress and negative energies being exhaled out of your system. You are getting cleansed with every breath.*

2. *If you want to take this meditation technique a step further, you can visualize inhaling positive energy. Think of a happy memory as you inhale and absorb the positive energy.*

3. *When you are ready to end this meditation, simply think of your physical body, move your fingers and toes, and slowly open your eyes, and affirm, "I am cleansed."*

This is a wonderful meditation technique since intermittent fasting is also a cleansing diet. While intermittent fasting, your body will reach the state of autophagy whereby it will eat away unhealthy cells and substances in the body.

Of course, this is only possible when you do not binge and eat unhealthy foods during your eating window. Remember that intermittent fasting is not only about not eating but it also about making healthy food choices if you want to experience the full benefits of this diet.

Indeed, when you are on an intermittent fast, the practice of regular meditation can be very helpful for you. The key to learning meditation is to practice it regularly. It is advised that you do it every day.

- **Drink Coffee, Tea, or Fresh Juice**

Many people who go on an intermittent fast allow the consumption of liquid beverages provided that they have 0 calories or at least a very low-calorie count.

However, if you want to experience the best benefits of this diet, it is advised that you only consume pure water during your fasting period. Still, there are many people who drink coffee and tea and even low-calorie fresh juice. This is a matter of personal preference for you to decide on. The problem with this is that coffee and tea can be acidic, depending on your body.

There are people who might suffer from an upset stomach if they drink coffee or tea without eating any solid food. This is another reason why drinking only water is recommended. The advantage of being able to consume other beverages, especially tea and coffee, is that it can help you feel full, and so you would not have to deal with too much with hunger. It is worth noting, however, that when you go on an intermittent fast, you would not have to worry so much about hunger once your body has adjusted to the diet.

- **Continuous Practice**

Learning intermittent fast is just like learning a new skill. This means that even while you may know what steps to take, you will most probably have to try it out several times before you can do it well. Take, for example, a person who wants to learn how to draw. Even if you give them a book on drawing, and even if they memorize it, they will most likely not be able to make a masterpiece right away.

Instead, they will have to practice for some time before they can do it well. The same is true when it comes to learning intermittent fasting. But, if you have a strong determination and willpower, you will probably be able to succeed on your first try. The idea here is to not give up and just keep on trying. This is a good way to make your body adjust and learn whatever it is that you want it to learn.

- **Cook Your Own Food**

To ensure that you will be eating high-quality and healthy foods, it is best to cook your own meals. This way, you will know exactly what ingredients are being mixed or used to prepare your dishes. Unfortunately, many foods, especially from fast-food chains, are unhealthy. So, you might want to prepare your own meals. This is also a good way to lower your expenses as it is usually cheaper to cook on your own than to buy ready-made foods.

If you are feeling confident, you might also want to try your hand on gardening and growing your own fresh fruits and vegetables. Research also shows that gardening is a relaxing activity. When you make your own food, primarily focus on natural foods like vegetables and fruits. Make it as organic as possible. As the saying goes, "You are what you eat." So according to this saying, you definitely want to put a lot of thought into what you are about to intake.

- **Stay Away from Temptations**

When you are just starting out, it is especially best to stay away from temptations as much as possible. Avoid going to places where you will be tempted to eat and break free from your diet during fasting hours. Every temptation presents another stress. You will want to lessen the stress that you feel as you fast. So, be mindful of your environment and the places that you go to. A good advice is just to stay home so that you are not lured to a restaurant. You should also be mindful of the people you hang out with.

For instance, instead of spending time with someone who loves to eat, hangout with someone who is also intermittent fasting or eating healthy. This way, you will be more motivated to succeed. Do not worry; this kind of preventive measure is only temporary. Once you get used to intermittent fasting, you will notice how all these preventive measures will come naturally to you. In fact, you will rarely even feel tempted to eat during fasting hours even if there is food in front of you. This is something that you will learn over time.

- **Keep Yourself Busy**

A common advice is to keep yourself busy. Take out time to do things you enjoy. This is an excellent way to make time pass quickly so that you can reach your eating-window. When you fasting, try not to think about how hungry you are or how tempted you are to eat. That will only make you feel worse about the situation. Instead, focus on something else. You see, hunger can only be a problem if you give it attention.

If you do not recognize it, then the feeling will pass easily. A good thing about this is that once hunger passes, it will take several hours for it to return. By that time, you can choose to ignore it again, or patiently wait for your eating-window time. However, if you continue to submit to those hunger pangs, you will become a slave to your own cravings, and you will not be able to enjoy the benefits of intermittent fasting.

- **Avoid Tiring Activities**

While it is perfectly safe to exercise while fasting, it is probably best you skip tiring activities. This will prevent you from feeling hungry. While exercising can make you feel good, you are likely to feel empty and hungry a few hours after you exercise.

So, for example, if you are on the Warrior Diet where you only eat in the evening, exercising in the morning can easily make you feel hungry in the afternoon. If you are not used eating, you are likely to find fasting a real challenge. But do not worry, with enough practice, you can exercise as much as you want and still not have a hard time sticking to your diet.

- **Use Positive Affirmations**

While intermittent fasting, you should maintain a positive mindset. One of the most effective ways to induce a positive mindset is by using affirmations. An affirmation is a statement that you tell yourself, usually repeatedly.

You are probably familiar with how this works. For example, when a person is feeling afraid, instead of admitting that they are afraid, they should affirm, "I am strong and courageous." The same technique can be used when you engage in intermittent fasting.

When using affirmations, you need to observe certain guidelines: First, the affirmation should be positive in nature. Hence, do not say that you cannot do something. Instead, be positive and say, "I am strong," or "I am patient," Or "I can do this," depending on the situation.

Feel free to make your own positive affirmation. It is also a good idea to keep your affirmation short and clear. It is advised that you limit your affirmation it to a single sentence. Next, you should believe and have fate in what you are about to say. If you do not believe in what you are about to say then it is unlikely to have an impact on you. You should also use present tense.

Using past tense may prevent something from happening while using future tense is no better because the future is always uncertain. Therefore, use present tense to declare your affirmation out loud. Now, there are no hard and fast rules on how many times you should repeat yourself. Just recite it to yourself as many times as you want when you feel like you need some push or encouragement, especially if there is no one else to motivate you.

Last but not least, you should believe that whatever you say has already happened or is already happening. Consider this as some kind of sleight of mind if you would. The more you believe it, the greater its chances of coming true.

- **Enjoy**

Since you will probably follow intermittent fasting for a long time, it is crucial you learn appreciate your journey. Many people who try this diet end up enjoying it after some time. This usually happens when you learn to appreciate the beauty of being healthy and your body starts adjusting to your new lifestyle.

Once you get the hang of it, you will find that intermittent fasting is actually a lot of fun. This is primarily why people continue this diet for long periods of time. As discussed, it is true that intermittent fasting is the kind of diet that you can practice for a long period, even for a lifetime. Unlike other diet programs that people often quit once they have lost weight, the IF diet can be followed for as long as you like.

The good news is that the more you practice intermittent fasting, the more you will get used to it, the easier it will get, and the healthier you will become.

- **Do not smoke**

Yes, not smoking is also a part of this section. Some people tend to smoke more often when they are fasting. This is quite harmful considering the side effects of smoking on one's health.

It should also be noted that intermittent fasting is not just about losing weight, but it is more about being healthy. And smoking does not quite fit the paradigm of being healthy. So, consider making an effort to stop smoking. If you cannot stop smoking right away, you can try gradually decreasing the number of cigarettes you smoke each day. The important thing to do here is to be healthy. At times, smoking can also trigger your urge to eat.

Of course, it is definitely not easy to quit smoking, but it is quite doable if you set your heart to it. If you honestly feel like you cannot drop this unhealthy habit and have already been enslaved by it, then it is only because you are yet to realize your inner strength and potential.

This is one of the nice things about intermittent fasting. It will not just encourage you to be healthier, but it will also make you realize your true strength – in turn, all of these things will add a positive change to your life.

- **Do not try too hard**

Trying too hard can be counterproductive as it will only buildup stress levels. Instead, just take it easy and. In fact, enjoy life. Intermittent fasting is very simple. The only challenge here is to be patient during fasting hours. Needless to say, you would not have any problems during the eating-window. As far as fasting is concerned, it is more about inaction and applying self-control. It is simply a matter of time.

Thankfully, since this is intermittent fasting, you do not have to wait for too long to reach your eating window. If you think of it this way, you will see that there is no reason at all for you to give yourself a hard time or take things too seriously. Just relax and enjoy life. If you feel like you cannot complete your fast and are already suffering too much, go ahead and break your fast and try again next time.

- **Gradual improvement**

You do not need to master intermittent fasting right away. Especially if you have never fasted before. Your new diet may shock your body in the beginning so try fasting every alternate day. Take note that you do not have to rush the learning process. In fact, it is advised that you take things slow and build yourself up gradually.

Hence, start with the 16/8 cycle, and then move forward to 23/1, and then alternate fasting. If you get used to alternate fasting, you might want to try fasting for two consecutive days. However, just remember to nourish your body properly.

Unlike regular fasting where you deliberately deprive your body of food and nutrients, intermittent fasting allows you to eat during your eating-window to help nourish your body. So, if you're feeling, remember to hang in there, this too will pass.

The Magic Of Water

Water is your best friend when you are intermittent fasting. Hence, it is only right for us to talk about it. Yes, we do believe that plain natural water is quite underrated. The human body can survive for many days without food, but not without water. In fact, most of the human body is composed of water, even our muscles.

Water is also the number one cleansing element of the body. If you want to cleanse your system, then drink lots of water every day. Many suggest that you should drink at least 8 cups of water to cleanse your system of toxins. It should be noted that this is the recommended average consumption. If you exercise, you will have to drink more than 8 glasses per day.

Now, if you are on fasting, you can drink more than 8 glasses. In fact, the more water you drink, the more you will be able to clean your body of impurities. When you encounter dreaded hunger pangs (which you surely will), you can drink water to feel full and satiated. Indeed, water is your best friend during these fasting periods. Of course, you can also drink coffee or tea, but the acid content might hurt your stomach. Also, if you completely want to cleanse your insides, then you should not drink any other beverage except water.

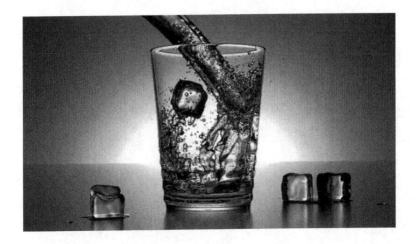

It is also a good practice to drink warm water early in the morning. It activates your digestive system and cleanses it. It also raises the temperature of the body, drastically increasing the fat-burning power of the body. Needless to say, water has zero calories, so it will never make you fat.

Most fail to drink enough water is because they don't keep water at hand. Hence, you might want to bring a bottle or portable container with you wherever you go to keep yourself hydrated. To know if you are well hydrated, inspect the color of your urine. If it is clear, it means that you are hydrated. If not, then you should immediately drink more water.

This is just one way to increase your daily water intake. You do not necessarily have to drink hot water. If you want, you can also drink cold water. The important thing is to drink lots of water to cleanse and hydrate your body.

If you want to avoid eating too much during your eating window, a good advice is to drink at least two glasses of water around 10 minutes before you eat. This way, you will feel quite full before you start eating and break your fast. If you fasting and have started to feel hungry, you can drink at least 3 glasses of water to curb hunger.

It is worth noting the difference between being truly hungry and feeling hungry. Most of the time, the body signals hunger, even when you are not in need of food. Understand that you are not really hungry, and are only feeling hungry at the moment.

In this case, drinking lots of water and simply letting the feeling pass on its own should be enough. Remember our rule when you fast: drink lots of water.

Do not confuse intermittent fasting with water fasting. Water fasting is when you do not eat at all or drink any other beverages except water. It is also not possible for someone to follow this fast for an extended period.

While intermittent fasting, you get an added benefit of cleansing your body of toxins and impurities, but you can use this diet for a lifetime, which is another reason why many people love intermittent fasting. After all, it is not easy to change one's eating habits again and again. If you take up intermittent fasting as a lifestyle, you will benefit from a healthy diet for as long as you live.

Chapter 5
Intermittent Fasting as A Way of Life

The Intermittent Fasting Lifestyle

Can intermittent fasting be considered as a lifestyle? Well, that depends. You see, the meaning of intermittent fasting will depend on what you make out of it. If you just see it as a way to regulate eating and fasting periods, then it is more like any other diet and not a lifestyle.

However, if you take it seriously and move a step further, where you do not only observe the window time but also follow the best practices in this book like living a healthy life and making healthier food choices, then intermittent fasting can be considered as a full-fledged lifestyle.

It is actually recommended that you view it more as a lifestyle. After all, it is safe to use this diet plan for as long as you want – and it is very good for you and your body. A common problem is to go on a healthy diet only to go back to being unhealthy after you have achieved desired results.

This is common for most diet plans out there where you follow a specific diet for a few weeks or months, only to leave it towards the end. After this, you will probably be left with no direction on what to do next, causing you to steer back to your regular unhealthy ways, which will only ruin everything that you have ever worked hard for.

With intermittent fasting, you do not have to deal with mere temporary benefits, as long as you make it your lifestyle. Yes, it will probably take some time before you can master it, but it is nonetheless doable, and you are the right person to do it.

To turn it into a lifestyle, you first have to get used to it. And the good news is that it is not really that difficult.

After all, unlike a regular fast where you will have to go without food for days and starve, intermittent fasting allows you to eat and soothe yourself during the eating-window – and this is a regular part of your routine. Also, if you are not aiming to take up alternate fasting or others, you can just stick to the usual 16/8 fast. It is actually very easy to get used to the 16/8 cycle.

The good news is that after a couple of days have passed, you can easily increase the number of fasting hours. Again, you do not have to rush the learning process. The important thing is to focus on quality and how well your body adjusts to the diet.

Indeed, if you want to get the most out of intermittent fasting, you need to turn it into a lifestyle. Of course, it does not mean that you will not get anything from it if you just use it for a few days. After all, the wonderful benefits of this diet are available to all of those who apply it in their lives.

As a lifestyle, this means that you would be used to the diet already. It should be noted that the 16/8 cycle is also considered as an intermittent fast. In fact, it is the most common IF cycle that you can find. So, if you want to quickly turn the IF diet into a lifestyle, you can simply master the 6/18 cycle. This is something that you can do in just a few weeks if you really give it your best shot. From there, it is up to you and whether or not you want to build up to a more intense cycle or not.

It is actually a blessing to embrace intermittent fating as a lifestyle. It is not supposed to be mundane lifestyle that is designed to make you suffer. It is, in fact, a wonderful way of life. If you truly want to live a healthy life and really feel healthy, then you will never go wrong with the IF diet.

Unlike other diet plans that will make you go weak and starve for days, the IF diet will make you feel good about your body. This is why many people who switch to intermittent fasting stop looking for other diet alternatives and stick to only this one.

As a lifestyle, the IF diet will definitely pave a way to a healthier and happier life. Of course, you will just have to adjust in the beginning, but it is all worth it. If you put your focus on it, you can even turn intermittent fasting into a lifestyle in just a month's time.

Intermittent fasting is a lifestyle that can create lots of positive changes in your life. What's more is that it will directly influence your health. Hence, you will surely appreciate just how beneficial it is for your body.

Of course, in the beginning, while you are still learning the diet, your body will require time to adapt to it, but this is only temporary. After the adjustment period, you can finally continue with your intermittent fast without any problems. So, what are you waiting for? It is time for you to make intermittent fasting as a lifestyle and start living a truly healthy life.

How To Socialize When You Are Fasting

People do not always think about it, but you might be surprised by just how much of your social life revolves around food. When people meet up, especially adults, there is almost always a need to have good food served on the table. It is as if you cannot see one another without eating. When you go on an intermittent fast, this is something you might have to overcome.

And, yes, you can expect to deal with this many times, so you better know your way out and get used to it. Of course, this does not mean you should avoid meeting your friends. When you are on an IF diet, you are free to see your friends as many times as you like.

However, to avoid abandoning your diet, you need to prepare yourself for the situation first. You can expect that while you may have friends who would further applaud and encourage you on your IF diet, there may also be those who would try to talk you out of it.

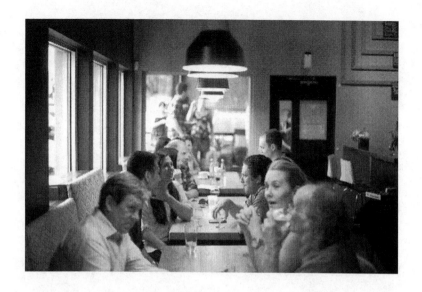

Remember that you do not have to argue or defend your position to anyone. Just remember why you started the diet in the first place and how it has helped you so far. This is where you need to make a firm stand and choose to stick to the IF diet.

This might be quite difficult in the beginning, but once you fully understand and appreciate the value of doing intermittent fasting, you would not be easily convinced or persuaded by other people to give it up.

Let us now discuss the real challenge: watching food being served in front of you, without being able to eat it. In such circumstances, it is best to take a deep breath and relax. I know it seems unfair and impossible, but there are many ways to deal with this.

Of course, the easiest would be to schedule your eating time window to coincide with the time you will be eating out with friends. Unfortunately, the problem is that this is not something that you can always rely on. Once you make intermittent fasting a crucial element of your lifestyle, you may at times find yourself feeling left out during dinner time with friends. So, what can you do? Well, while this is indeed challenging, it is something that you need to overcome.

This is the best time to consume drinks that have zero calories such as coffee and tea. Of course, you should also hydrate yourself well by drinking lots of water. You can also remind yourself that you are meeting your friends to spend time with them. You do not have to eat or do anything else except talk and chill out. This way, you will be more able to focus on your friends instead of allowing food to divide your attention. If you are a busy person and seldom get time to meet your friends, do not allow food to act as a barrier for you as intermittent fasting gets easier over time.

You should realize that socializing is about being with people and not about eating. This eating culture has only become popular in the modern world where everyone always feels the need to eat. However, this is exactly what intermittent fasting is all about: it teaches you to adapt a healthy lifestyle and not be controlled by society. This is a decision that you have to make; and more importantly, you have to stick to it.

Okay, when you do this, you can expect your friends to raise eyebrows and ask many questions. In this situation, many folks simply prefer to lie and say they are still full to avoid talking about the diet. However, it is best to just be honest about it and tell them the truth: Tell them all about intermittent fasting. Do not hesitate to share your experiences about the diet. In fact, you will find this approach more beneficial for you as you will no longer have to hide what you are feeling. If you are with positive people, then chances are that you will even feel more motivated to continue your diet. However, just a word of caution, if you are with people whom you know tend to be negative or discouraging, then it is best to just keep quiet and not talk about your diet.

Although when you do open up to people about your IF diet, keep in mind that you do not have to explain yourself to them. So, if you encounter someone who is against the idea simply, let them be. After you have explained your side, you do not have to do anything more. It is up to them whether they will believe you or not. They are not your problem. Your only obligation is to stick to your diet and enjoy its wonderful benefits. You do not have to prove this to anyone.

Conclusion

Thanks for making it through to the end of this eBook. I hope you found this book informative and were able to benefit from the guidelines mentioned to achieve your goals, whatever they may be.

The next step is to apply everything that you have learned and start enjoying the benefits of intermittent fasting. Remember that being healthy is a choice and your diet should be a way of life. By now, you are already armed with the right knowledge and tools about intermittent fasting. As you already know, acquiring knowledge alone is not enough. You also need to turn it into practice.

As a beginner, kindly expect that the initial stages can be difficult, especially when you are not used to fasting. To make it easier for you, do it gradually. You do not have to rush and jump to a 16-hour fast right away. Once again, you need to focus on the quality of learning.

The more you are able to adjust and master this diet, the easier it will become for you, in turning it into a lifestyle.

Unlike other diet plans, it is recommended you consider intermittent fasting as a lifestyle rather than a temporary diet program to lose weight. This is primarily why the IF diet is designed to last a lifetime, simply because it is meant to be practiced for life.

This book has given you all the keys you need to stay healthy. It is now up to you to apply everything that you have learned and live a healthy and happier life.

Finally, if you have found this eBook useful in anyway, a review on Amazon is always appreciated!

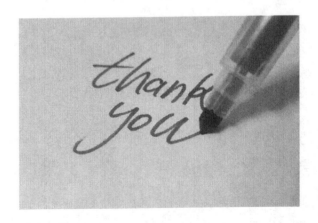

11288422R00073

Made in the USA
Lexington, KY
09 October 2018